Free Bonus Fc

Information needed by Dementia caregivers is on the internet but how do you find it quickly? I spend hours reviewing sites and here is your solution!!!

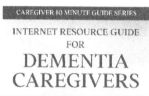

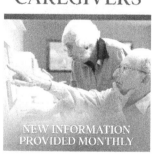

- **Websites**

- **Podcasts**

- **Blogs**

- **Virtual Support Groups**

Caregivers don't have time to research, so I did it for you. And as an additional gift, new sites of interest will be distributed whenever a valuable source of information for the dementia caregiver is discovered...ALL FREE!

Join the private Caregiver 10 Minute Guides mailing list to download this free book. I promise no spam or sale of this list.

www.Caregiver10minuteguides.com

The 10 Minutes Caregiver Guides

Time is precious, and never more so than for caregivers. Information is needed in a concise manner that can be absorbed quickly and immediately offer solutions to problems. This is the goal of all *Caregiver 10 Minute Guides*.

Book 1:

Visiting with Love: Productive Activities for Memory and Elder Care Residents

Book 2:

Communicating with Love: Creating Joyful Conversations with Memory Care and Elder Care Residents

Future Topics include:

- Behavioral Issues of Alzheimer and Dementia Residents

- Long Distance Caregiving
- End of Life Issues for Alzheimer and Dementia Residents

Visiting with Love: Productive Activities for Memory and Elder Care Resident

The 10 Minute Caregiver Guide Series

Published by CAREShare

Copyright © 2021 by E. Jane Wyatt

ISBN: 9798598951477

Dedication

There are too many people to acknowledge who have encouraged, pushed, and stood for me over the years. It's a good thing I plan to do a series of books. I can continue to express my gratitude over multiple volumes and maybe include everyone.

But for this first book:

Joyce Fox...you opened the door that led me to find my passion.

DuAnne Redus...I had shut that door. You held on to the vision of me opening it again.

Bev Nykamp and Karen Moore...thanks for keeping my ADD personality moving forward. And for always believing.

Of course, I must mention the greatest inspiration in my life, my Mother. I did not have most of these suggestions available when I was visiting her so I was left to do the best I could. In her memory, I share with you the ideas I wish I had known.

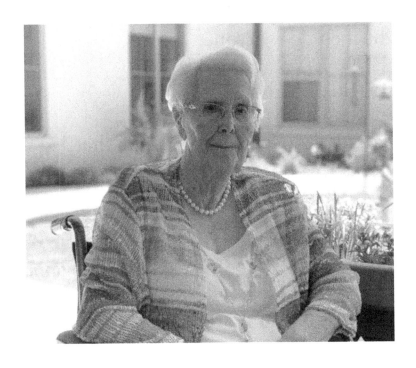

Lorene J. Murphy

June 24, 1921 – April 14, 2020

Visiting with Love

Productive Activities for Memory Care and Elder Care Residents

Introduction

I admit that this book was born out of anger.

The anger that motivated this book came from the reality that many of the people my mom had spent her life with, especially her church family, practically abandoned her in those final days.

When she was finally committed to a memory care facility, I expected people would take time to visit her and lift her spirits. But she didn't have many visitors. It was only when I could admit to myself that visiting someone you love that has mentally left you, is really difficult. I came to realize that Mom's friends and family didn't know how to visit. They didn't know what to do on a visit that left all feeling good.

Visiting someone in memory care is extremely hard; it also presents various challenges. It is difficult to visit a person who does not remember who you are and has few or no memory of any time before that minute. Yet you will reap great rewards from visits to your loved one and friend.

This book discusses what I have learned about preparing for time spent with a resident of a memory care center. I also offer suggestions on preparing activities that can assist in a productive interaction.

Contents

Chapter 1: What To Know (and Do) Before You Visit

"You get out what you put in. If you want more, give more"

Jeanette Jenkins

Let's be clear about the goals for this book. When you are with a memory impaired person, you want them to feel your affection. You want them engaged and comforted by being the focus of your attention. Your goal will be deemed successful with their smile and allowing them a little bit of sunshine.

What is the goal for yourself? To leave the memory care center feeling that your time was well-spent. The person you visited was only a hint of the individual you once knew. By visiting, you honor the past you once shared. You radiate love and friendship to the person they have become, knowing this change was thru no fault of their own.

Like any other task, preparation is the key to success. You must be willing to invest time understanding what could encourage interest from the resident. You need to be ready to lead conversations and activities appropriate to their physical and mental abilities.

Below are recommendations on what that preparation might entail.

Do your research

When a loved one is in a memory care facility, the chances are high that they may not consciously remember what pastimes they used to enjoy. Perhaps they had playful hobbies like Karaoke, darts, yoga, pottery, makeup, or stamp collecting. Just because they don't remember these hobbies doesn't mean they wouldn't enjoy them if you suggested it.

If you don't know exactly what someone likes to spend their time on, do your research by talking to family or other friends. Ask if there are special songs or types of music they enjoy. Did the resident like to cook? What was their favorite recipe? Is there anything that might trigger a memory for them and bring the happiness of something familiar?

Prepare for Groundhog Day

In the 1993 iconic film, Groundhog Day, Bill Murray's character, Phil, repeatedly lives the same day.

The lives of patients at memory care centers are intentionally structured to feel like they are reliving the same day repeatedly. That's why the staff at these facilities have nicknamed this process Groundhog Day.

When your loved one has a memory capacity that deteriorates with each passing day, they need repetition, structure, and routine to stay emotionally and mentally balanced.

Most people find a persistent routine too boring, but for a patient with dementia, a routine is calming and reassuring. Therefore, before you visit, ask either the staff or the primary caregiver the best days and/or times of the day to visit. What time are meals served? Allowing the memory-impaired person to maintain their routine is important.

Your visit provides a special value.

Most memory care centers proudly advertise activity programs for their residents. There will probably be a person designated as the Activities Director. It might be felt that the center offers plenty of socialization opportunities. Another misconception is that when the resident struggles to remember what happened an hour ago, it is futile to spend time with that person. After all, they may not even recall your visit.

Here's the truth:

Just because your loved one may not remember that you visited them doesn't negate the visit's value. When you spend time with a loved one in a memory care center and make the person smile, although they may lose the memory of the experience, they will not lose the health and emotional benefits of experiencing positive interactions.

Having organized activity sessions is certainly positive. But let's be realistic. The staff at care facilities is often overworked or slow in their duties. That is certainly understandable when you consider that the staff oversees everything: meals, hygiene, laundry, medication and so on. Most often, the activity hour is a group filled with individuals at different stages of dementia, both physically and mentally. Often the activity is conducted by a staff member who is thinking about the tasks they still have to do instead of stimulating individual interaction. Although conducted with the best of intentions, the staff can't meet the needs of all residents.

Your visit is the greatest source of stimulation for residents of a memory care facility. Your individual is receiving focused direct attention. The resident may quickly lose the memory of the visit, but the general sense of being appreciated and loved will remain long after you depart.

- ## *Be adaptive to their moods*

Unpredictable emotional states are one of the symptoms of dementia. When you visit your loved one, you must understand the importance of being flexible. Your ability to be a good companion will rest a lot on reading their mood and adapting. I frequently teach that the purpose of your visit is to join their reality.

I walked into the center one day and saw a resident who was obviously sad. It was unusual because Judith was normally perky and very social. I sat down to talk to her, and she tearfully told me that her mother was dying. Did I mention that Judith was in her 90's? Obviously, her belief wasn't true.

In this situation, the most beneficial path was to validate her feelings. I expressed how sorry I was to hear such bad news. I then began to ask questions about her mother and encourage Judith to share memories with me. Gently, I tried to lead to sharing funny and happy stories about her mother and family.

If today your loved one wants a shoulder to cry on, be there for them, and if tomorrow they want to laugh, have a good joke ready. Be in their reality.

- ***Carry an assortment of gear with you***

It's a great idea to carry a tote bag containing items related to activities your loved one enjoys. In the following chapters are multiple suggestions for things to bring with you. Having a variety of such objects ensures a visit that both of you will enjoy.

- ***Read up on the symptoms (to ensure nothing catches you by surprise)***

Dementia is a general term that encompasses illnesses that result in loss of memory, language problems, inability to focus, and difficulty solving problems.

Alzheimer's disease, vascular dementia, Lewy Body Disease, and Front-temporal dementia all fall under dementia, but their causes and progression can differ.

Taking time to understand the progression and resulting symptoms of the illness is a necessary step that helps you understand why your loved one is acting a specific way.

Here are some symptoms to keep in mind:

Early dementia symptoms:

- Confusion

- Difficulty concentrating

- Depression

- Withdrawal

- Communication problems

Advanced dementia symptoms:

- Difficulty moving

- Needing help with hygiene and self-care

- Difficulty swallowing

- Inability to speak

- Complete forgetfulness

In concluding this chapter, the key to a happy engagement is taking the time to invest in knowledge of your loved ones' well-being. Preparing your visit based on research on activities most likely to trigger engagement and happiness. Determining the best time and day to visit. Knowing a little about the common symptoms of Alzheimer's and dementia.

Thinking in advance about your options for making the visit a good one for both of you.

In the next chapter, I discuss how physical contact plays a huge role in caring for a loved one in a memory care facility.

Chapter 2: The Magic of Touch

"The human touch is that little snippet of physical affection that brings a bit of comfort, support, and kindness. It doesn't take much from the one who gives it, but can make a huge difference in the one who receives it."

Mya Robarts

While writing this book in 2020, the world has been focused on the significant death toll and illness created by COVID-19. In every conversation whether family, friends, or complete strangers, a sentiment has been expressed universally. *"I miss hugs"* is the common lament offered by so many. Social distancing is a sensible response to a pandemic that transmits through proximity, but I hope it taught us a valuable lesson. *We should never take holding or touching each other for granted.* It is amazing how much joy comes from a hug, or a simple pat.

Multiple experiments have been conducted since World War II to determine if human touch truly has health benefits. Studies more recently have included using MRI and Cat Scans to differentiate types of brain activity between when the subject was touched or had no contact. Scientists discovered that when we are touched in a caring method, the body releases the major hormones of dopamine, oxytocin, serotonin, and endorphins transmitting chemical reactions within the body activating feelings of well-being and mood stabilization.

Following are touch activities you can engage in when you visit your loved one.

Massage

Almost everyone enjoys a good massage, but for individuals suffering from cognitive problems, this could be their saving grace. Unlike memories, which the mind may be quick to forget, the body does not forget the positive effects of receiving a nice shoulder rub. Research conducted on dementia patients in care facilities and published in the National Institute of Health[1] found that hand massages with oil helped reduce agitation behavior amongst patients.

---

[1] https://www.ncbi.nlm.nih.gov/pmc/articles/PMC6223738/

As a retired massage therapist, I would like to offer these suggestions.

- **A soothing atmosphere**

As with most activities with a memory impaired resident, it is preferable to spend your visit time in a location free from distractions. Consider playing some soothing music to create a peaceful atmosphere.

- **Use oil or lotion**

Using a small amount of lotion creates a sliding motion that reduces friction and increases pleasurable sensations. Consider using an oil or lotion that has a fragrant aroma to add to the enjoyment of the touch.

- **Rub gently**

Use your fingers to rub the target area in gentle circles. Massage the skin and muscles. Applying pressure on the bones is not pleasurable to anyone, especially seniors. Use a firm, gentle, slow action for the best results.

Playdough

As a child, you might have played with this material; thus, it should be easy to do it again now. If you are unfamiliar with it, here is the gist of it. Playdough is a fun activity where you use a thick, elastic, and malleable material to make different shapes and structures.

The mere act of kneading is good for stimulating parts of the brain responsible for hand to eye coordination, and thus, dementia patients gain a lot from it. It is possible to play with playdough alone, but you can work on it together to increase physical touch between you and your loved one. Creating innovative structures together while stimulating the sense of touch will be good for your loved one's mental and physical well-being.

Here are some tips if you decide to integrate playdough into your activities with a memory-afflicted loved one:

- **Take advantage of nasal sensory awareness**

A fun fact to know is that the brain associates memory far more strongly with smell than sight or sound. Psychotherapists often use smell to trigger suppressed memories. By adding essential oil or food extracts to the molding clay, you may create strong pleasurable memories. You can easily find internet recipes to add scent to the dough.

- **Cookie cutters can stimulate play**

Include fun shaped cookie cutters in your visiting kit to stimulate conversation and play with the playdough. It is recommended that you use a cookie sheet or wax paper to protect the table surface.

Manicures and Brushing Hair

Most people love to be pampered, such as a manicure or having your hair styled. The resident in a memory care facility gets the same uplift in spirits when given personal attention. For the caregiver, it is not expected that you would perform the same perfection achieved by a nail care technician. Tasks such as cutting nails should be left to trained professionals. The objective here is to create a soothing, fun activity. Use a warm cloth to wash the hands. Incorporate a hand massage as described previously with a pleasant-smelling lotion. Let the resident pick the color of the fingernail polish. Brush their hair with gentle strokes. And most important, compliment the resident on their groomed appearance.

Hand Puppets and Stuffed Toys

The value of therapy animals is another professionally researched and established practice. It has been shown many times over that stroking the fur or playing with the animals lessens confusion and projects pleasurable feelings. Did you know that the sense of touch is so desired that stuffed toys can create a similar reaction? Or for a more interactive activity, use finger and hand puppets. It's easy to promote a fun pastime that encourages touch and communication and hopefully...some silliness.

Chapter 3: The Mood-Altering Effect of Music

"Where words fail, music speaks."

Hans Christian Andersen

When driving to work, I listen to music on the radio to get me pumped up and ready for the day. For my evening drive, I have a different type of music signaling that it is time to begin unwinding from the hectic day. There is nothing in the world that is as effective at changing our mood as listening to music. The human brain responds to music differently than it does to noise or speech.

A study conducted by the University College London confirmed the benefits of music. Their research documented that the brain responds to music by increasing cognitive speeds to an above-average range. Further when the brain hears music it releases dopamine, a neurotransmitter responsible for positive emotions.

The research into the benefits of music for Alzheimer or dementia patients is especially worth noting. It has been proven that the key areas of the brain that store musical memory are relatively undamaged during the progression of these diseases. Which in turn means that a music relationship, in any form, may outlast all other memory functions. The benefits of music for dementia patients include:

- Reducing stress

- Eliminating depression

- Reducing agitation

So, playing music during your visit may create a special connection. The sounds can help your loved one relax and to improve their mood. The purpose is not your enjoyment; it's for the enjoyment of your loved one! Choose the music based on their preferences. If playing a particular song agitates them, switch to another tune. Likewise, note their favorite songs to play for them again in the future.

Here are suggestions for including music on your visit.

Play songs that also have movement involved

I recall watching an Alzheimer's patient named Ginger uproariously do "The Chicken Dance" totally without instruction or prompts. It was so embedded in her memory that she was teaching other residents to do the dance. There was such joy and laughter for her and others as she performed the hand and body actions associated with that music.

Many other songs also have a dance or fun hand gestures to imitate. You can easily find suggests on the internet and YouTube. As you are singing and doing the dance with the memory impaired individual, a sense of connection gives you the same feeling of playfulness and creates a fun memory for your future.

Here are a few fun song suggestions:

- *The Itsy Bitsy Spider*

- *The Hokey Pokey*

- *Down By the Old Mill Stream*

- *The Wheels on the Bus*

- *If You're Happy and You Know It*

Let them play a musical instrument

Having a personal "noisemaker" encourages creative expression and participation. Children's toys can supply an inexpensive source of drums, tambourines, or even piano keyboards. It could also be as simple as putting dry beans or pennies in a tightly sealed plastic container to shake to the beat.

Customize the music played

In the first chapter of this book, it was recommended that you prepare in advance by remembering or investigating the preferences of the resident. Remember to find music your loved one likes. Find who their favorite musicians are. If no one knows what the resident likes, experiment by playing the top playlist from different decades and watch their response.

Sing along Music

It is not important if anyone remembers the words to a song. Yet having a lyric song sheet adds a kinesthetic component to the activity and allows others to participate. There are many sources on the internet to download or purchase playlists of sing-along music. Many elders will relate to the 1960's musical variety show of "Sing Along with Mitch" and the instructions to "follow the bouncing ball" as the words to the song were displayed on the screen. Please remember that any good experience is always better when you share it with someone. Having you around will boost their mood and create a stronger mental association.

Dance

In the second chapter, we noted that the sense of touch is a powerful tool that can help calm a person down and form a bond with them. Imagine what would happen if you combined the power of music and touch to help relax a loved one's mind and create a strong bond.

Dancing may be one of the most powerful things you might instigate for residents in a memory care center. You can even dance with someone in a wheelchair by just holding their hands and swaying in time with the music.

Consider calming classical or religious pieces

There will be times when the music you play is focused on creating a calm environment. Perhaps the resident is agitated. Or maybe your visit is shortly before they retire to sleep. Music may be used for distraction and to de-escalate tension. Beethoven's *Moonlight Sonata* or Tchaikovsky's *Hymn of the Cherubim* are great pieces to try out. Classical music pieces are some of the most cathartic because they directly affect brain waves. For the resident who was previously involved in a church, it may be particularly soothing to hear songs of their faith.

Chapter 4: The Joy of Accomplishment

"Joy, feeling one's own value, being appreciated and loved by others, feeling useful and capable of production are all factors of enormous value for the human soul."

Maria Montessori

We all want to feel appreciated and valued, to know that we're capable of doing a task and receiving praise when we do it well. Our care recipients are no different.

No adult wants to feel managed or spoken to in a condescending manner. At some level, our care recipients have felt their basic capabilities of structure and reason slipping away. The mental and physical demise brings a loss of independence because they can no longer care for themselves. In a short time, the feelings of uselessness and depression become all too common.

Fortunately, with just a little thought and imagination on your part, you can change that impression. While you know that you could do a task faster and better, focus instead on the gift you are giving your loved one by allowing them to participate in failure-free activities.

Perhaps your loved one cannot assist in the kitchen or cut up vegetables, but they could stir the dry ingredients. The task does not even have to have any importance beyond giving the care recipient a sense of purpose and an opportunity to receive praise and appreciation.

Here are a few steps you can take:

Allow them to take care of their body needs

Self-grooming is a very personal affair, and by undertaking this process on someone else's behalf, it is possible to make them feel like a child.

Let your memory-handicapped loved one clean his/her face, comb their hair, apply their makeup, wash their body and brush their teeth. Letting someone accomplish these tasks for themselves will give them a sense of control over their own lives. That is important because as their mind starts to fail them, they will need activities that make them feel competent and capable.

Just because you want to encourage independence does not mean you should be careless. Always keep a watchful eye to avoid falls or contact with unsafe items.

When my mother was in the early stages of dementia, I started noticing that her time in the shower was 3 minutes or less. Obviously not sufficient time to get a good body wash. Directly addressing the issue only brought the attitude of "I'll do it myself" as she considered assistance in the shower a reflection of her loss of ability and independence. At last, I was able to negotiate a compromise. Mom loved to have her back rubbed, and I started by remarking that I bet it was hard for her to wash her own back. Once I could assist with the back wash, it was simple to expand to the legs and other body areas. But I would also give her the washcloth and insist that she wash the front of her body and private parts. In that manner, we both achieved our objectives without loss of dignity.

Encourage simple chores

We all have a deep-seated need to engage in productive activities. Chores are a great way to provide an outlet for this desire to be useful. As I write this, I'm smiling because of the irony of how the most tedious household chores become golden moments for the Alzheimer/dementia care recipients. Folding laundry, which I don't enjoy, is a prize to the person that wants so much to feel helpful.

The chores can be simple and failure-free. Jobs like polishing silver, folding towels, sweeping the floor, or polishing shoes can give the memory impaired individual the delight of feeling productive.

Gardening activities

Tending to a garden is rather symbolic of looking after a child. From the act of planting new life and working with nature, there can be a lot of pride in working on this kind of project. The garden can be flowers for aesthetic purposes or a food garden providing the ultimate reward of getting to eat what is grown. The repetition of visiting the garden each day to survey new growth allows a wonderful opportunity for interactive conversation.

Making jewelry or other forms of craftwork

Throughout this chapter, information that has been shared should give a good foundation for evaluating safe activities. With that knowledge, a short walk through a hobby store or exploring online sites will provide multiple suggestions for appropriate craft activities. Indeed, many crafts come in complete kits with all material included. I discovered fleece tie kits. Mom was able to tie the simple knot and enjoyed the textile feel of the material. Finishing gave her a sense of pride.

I want to reiterate an important point. The success of these activities is not dependent on if the project is finished or how well it is done. Seriously, is any of that really important? If it is, you should be doing the craft yourself.

The wise Maya Angelou said: "At the end of the day people won't remember what you said or did, they will remember how you made them feel. This has an element of truth even for the memory impaired. The importance of your visit is the love communicated to those whose world has shrunk so drastically.

Now that you understand the importance of accomplishing tasks, the next chapter delves into the health benefits of physical movement.

Chapter 5: The Power of Movement

"Movement is a medicine for creating change in a person's physical, emotional, and mental states."

Carol Welch

There is so much research needed for dementia and Alzheimer's. In my opinion, there was a delay in focusing on these debilitating diseases. "Senility" was too long accepted as an inevitable result of old age. Progress, however slowly it appears to be moving, is advancing treatment and prevention.

Not surprisingly a prime factor in the prevention and treatment of countless other diseases has once again been identified as a deterrent to dementia. The simple remedy of exercise/physical movement is showing results in preventing the onset and delaying the progression of dementia. In the November 2020 issue of Practical Neurology, doctors reviewed enough evidence of the neuroprotective effect of physical and cognitive activity to recommend it for patients. Their research indicated that physical activity alone or in combination with other interventions may protect and/or prevent cognitive decline and loss of function.

Most people engaged in physical activity have some sort of planned schedule. Perhaps they go for a jog each morning after awakening. Or they attend classes at a gym on a consistent day and time. The memory-impaired resident is probably not capable of self-directed exercise. Therefore, encouraging movement is very dependent on the caregiver or visitors.

Of course, we are not necessarily talking about a gym routine or jogging path that you might follow. Instead, we are referring to games or walks or dances which can not only increase cardiovascular health, but also supply additional benefits. For the Alzheimer's or dementia patient, physical activity has been found to reduce depression which is commonplace in memory care centers.

Exercise can also decrease restlessness and wandering, a widespread problem among memory care residents. Medical experts have noted that roaming often worsens when an Alzheimer's patient is restricted and has no change in scenery. While the familiar is comforting to the patient, the brain also craves seeing different places. Exploring different views, whether inside or out, while meandering with you allows them to feel safe while activating their childlike curiosity.

Walking and simple activities also assist in maintaining balance and improving coordination.

The success of any endeavor including physical activity will depend on your attitude as you engage in these activities. If your loved one senses your disinterest, then they too will lose interest, but if they sense your determination, then they will be more engaged. As the expression goes: Emotions are contagious.

Another pillar of success is offering physical activities the resident will enjoy. While one person will enjoy a walk in the sun, another person may prefer a game of mini golf. It's up to you to pay attention and anticipate what your loved one will engage in with pleasure.

Here are a few activities beneficial to memory care residents:

Balloon Volleyball

Balloon volleyball is as simple as possible because all you need is an extra-large balloon or beach ball.

Depending on the participants' mental and physical wellness, you can play it in teams with a net dividing the sides. You can also arrange those in wheelchairs in a circle and challenge them to keep the ball in the air while passing it to each other.

Whether as a group or a one-on-one activity, this game encourages movement, flexibility, and focused attention.

Going for a walk

Walking is ideal because it provides two simultaneous benefits. The first is improving physical health, and the second is allowing a change of scenery that the brain desperately needs. Consider providing tactile elements such as touching the tree bark or smelling a flower.

Games

Games involving throwing cornhole bean bags and rings are all playable using inexpensive and easily available equipment. They also allow participation from all including those fully mobile and those in wheelchairs.

I have heard of successful participation by utilizing an electronic program such as the Wii or a Playbox. They offer a variety of games such as bowling without the need of the actual equipment.

Stretching and Chair Exercises

You can encourage your loved one to engage in a daily stretching routine. Bending backward, forward, and sideways are all great ways to ensure that the muscles in the abdomen, back, and legs get adequate exercise. Stretching also improves coordination and balance while increasing blood flow. Stretching is great because it is easy to do without being too hard on the body.

In recent years, books, internet programs and DVD's teaching exercise performed while sitting at a desk has been made popular due to the increasing number of people working at computers. Many of these routines are appropriate for those in wheelchairs or challenged with balance. Review the information before attempting it with your memory care resident to confirm that the pace and routines are appropriate. And remember to enthusiastically join in the exercise.

The final chapter challenges us to practice mindfulness when we are visiting the memory care residents.

Chapter 6: The Intimacy of Being Present

"Making one person smile can change the world--maybe not the whole world, but their world."

Author unknown

The greatest present you can give a dementia patient is the gift of being truly present when you are with them. The term mindfulness has become popular in our culture. By definition, mindfulness is the mental state achieved by focusing one's awareness on the present moment.

Instead of thinking of your shopping list when you are at the facility, be genuinely connected and give direct eye contact. Listen intently, even if the words make no sense. Put down your cell phone and focus on letting your heart and affection show. After all, what value is a visit if done with a sense of obligation?

My Pet Peeve

I am invoking one of the benefits of being the author: the right to insert my own opinion. It is my belief that watching television with a dementia patient is a frequently abused activity forced on the memory impaired. Most of the time, television is simply hiding the fact that the visitor has spent no time preparing or has no interest in visiting. Even staff will prop dementia patients in front of a screen with the television blaring, believing it keeps them occupied and engaged. In reality, and from personal experience, most patients fall asleep with nothing accomplished.

With my next statement you may wonder what stage of dementia I am in because it is going to seem that I am contradicting myself. Watching television with a dementia patient can be a great activity provided it is done with the right intent and a strong degree of flexibility.

Watching a game in the World Series may please you but give the dementia resident little pleasure. But a classic TV show such as *I Love Lucy* might bring back a memory or inspire laughter. Watching a movie and even a musical may surprise you when the receiver begins singing along. Participate! Watch the show and interact, clap, comment, laugh, and ask questions with no wrong answers.

Additional suggestions:

- When looking for television shows or movies, consider the public library as a source of free DVD's.

- It is perfectly normal for the receiver to lose interest after a while. Expect this, accept this, and be ready to go to the next activity. If you get irritated because the person wants to move on before the show/movie is over, reexamine your own agenda about why you are visiting.

Play a game

It is unlikely that the memory-impaired resident can process a board game like Monopoly or chess. Strategy games may remind your loved one of the mental abilities they no longer have and create a sense of bewilderment or distress.

However, checkers or the ageless Chutes and Ladders game can spark great satisfaction from social interaction and stimulating mental connections. I have a great photo of Mom playing checkers with me. The checker "board" was made of fabric. And the pieces were super-sized for easy handling. It is a happy memory recalling her total glee and delight in beating me!

Additional suggestions:

- Colorful playing boards and large game pieces can be highly beneficial. When playing dominos or a card game, the special holder trays allow the player to participate more easily.

- Keep it simple. My sister created a great game by explaining that she needed to make certain that all the cards in a playing deck were there before she could start a game. She got Mom to sort the cards into suits and then put each suit in numerical order. And had Mom name each card while she was sorting. So simple, but it gave Mom a sense of purpose and accomplishment.

- Games with a time component are not helpful because they add an element of unneeded stress.

- The electronic games loved by children and teens today may seem extremely easy to operate yet be too much of a challenge to a dementia-afflicted loved one.

- Bingo is a popular game in memory care facilities. It promotes socializing and encourages focus and cognition.

- The old saying that "rules are made to be broken" should especially apply when playing games with dementia patients. The exact rules for any game do not matter. Add the satisfaction of giving the winner a prize, and although I know I do not have to suggest this, ensure that everybody wins!

Prepared conversation

The person who visits a dementia patient with the goal of "just talking about whatever the patient wants" will leave feeling disappointed. You could run out of conversation in five minutes or less if you are expecting them to initiate. Recognize the tiny little world of the dementia patient.

There is a misconception that speaking about the past may be stressful to the dementia patient. Dementia patients usually remember the distant past much more vividly than recent events. They may feel quite comfortable talking about things or people from long ago. Of course, the memory care resident may not remember that the event or person is in the past. And it is not your duty to correct them. Your purpose is to join them in their reality, not make them wrong.

At the very least, have a list of questions or topics to bring up. Ask questions that your loved one can answer with a yes or no. Follow with appropriate questions about the topic.

Here's an example: "Did you like to swim when you were young?" Was your favorite, swimming in a lake or the ocean? There are versions of the classic game "Twenty Questions" available for purchase on the internet. A set of those question cards could be a handy addition to your visiting tote bag.

Give enough time for an answer. Every minute does not have to be full of sound; your presence is a more important factor. Do not interrupt. Listen as though you have never heard the story before because the sad truth is it might be the last time you hear that version of the tale.

Read a book

There may be a time when your loved one is beyond verbal communication. That certainly does not mean that the person cannot benefit from the attention your visit brings. At other times, you may have scheduled a visit during their "active" time, only to find out that they want to stay in bed. That's a great time to read a book out loud. The soothing sound of your voice will bring a wonderful sense of calm and love.

What type of books? That will differ with each situation and person. The book may be on a hobby or career in which the patient participated. My grandfather was a railroad engineer, so I would have taken a book about trains to show him.

What we call "coffee table books" might be a good choice as they normally have large photos and limited text. Encourage your loved one to sit beside you, sharing their thoughts about each photo.

Go through photo albums with your loved one. Be ready for the experience to transport them to the past, and they may ask questions such as "That's Momma. When will she be coming home tonight?" In some instances, they may not even recognize themselves; that's okay too. Focus on the joy of being present with them.

Jigsaw puzzles

A simple pleasure for a dementia patient is to work and complete a jigsaw puzzle, especially as a shared activity. In addition to the accomplishment, the activity also improves manual dexterity and spatial skill.

- Choose a puzzle appropriate to the patient's cognitive functionalities. For some people, a 30–60 piece puzzle may be realistic. For others in a more advanced stage, the puzzle may need to be in the range of 6-15 pieces.

- Choose puzzles with simple images and large pieces. Colorful and pieces with well-defined corners add to the ease of working the jigsaws.

- In the late stages of my mother's dementia, I created a simple block puzzle out of a family photo that only had six pieces. Beyond the puzzle aspect, it allowed her to share her thoughts about each person in the picture.

Look at old photographs

As previously mentioned, a beautiful activity is going through photo albums or however you store past photos with your loved one. As their memories continue to fade, it is up to you to remind them that they had a wonderful life. Looking at old photos of their wedding day, their first car, their children and grandchildren is a great way to have fun and keep memories active in their minds.

They say a picture is worth a thousand words. Thus, it is far better to look at photos rather than only talking about memories. The moment will be more powerful when shared; participate in the act of looking at the pictures.

Tips to keep in mind:

- If you notice that a memory has slipped out of your loved one's conscious awareness, do not push the issue. Move on to another photo keeping the experience fun and stress free.

- Alzheimer's patients often remember older memories far better than newer ones. If you can find nice photos from their youthful years, reminiscing may be an enjoyable experience for your loved one.

Conclusion

I hope that the suggestions presented make your visits a happier occasion for both you and the person you visit.

According to data from Alzheimers.net,[2] more than 5 million Americans live with Alzheimer's, and by 2050, experts predict that this number will have tripled to 16 million. 1 in 3 seniors die with some form of Alzheimer's, and every 60 seconds, someone new develops the condition.

I bring up this data to help you understand that you are not alone; millions of people like you are looking after their parents, grandparents, relatives, and friends with these conditions.

I urge you to join CAREShare on Facebook, or to find another source of support. Some place where you can discuss your experiences with others in similar situations. Ask questions. Reveal feelings. Perhaps you have discovered a wonderful activity for the memory impaired. Share it with the group or anyone that may find it helpful. No matter what you learn or how you learn it, share. Your bit of wisdom could be the answer to someone else's prayer.

Because with complete certainly I can tell you:

---

[2] https://www.alzheimers.net/resources/alzheimers-statistics

Whatever you are feeling, you are not alone

Blessings on you, my dear caregiver.

About the Author

After sixty-odd years of pursuing various careers and interests, I was blessed to "find myself" once again. Twenty years earlier, I had been a hospice and mental health counselor and loved what I was doing. But as too often happens, life got in the way and I made the decision to leave that field. You might say that I put all my notes and books and indeed even my soul into storage.

Until in late 2020 I was led to believe that my personal legacy project wasn't to hide my knowledge but to put it into action. And with that, I started the creation of CAREShare: promoting Caregiving, Advocacy, Education, and Support. The first focus is on writing books under the series title Caregiver 10 Minute Guides. I am also active as a public speaker on visitation to dementia residents and assisting religious organizations with improvement with their ministry to the sick programs.

I appreciate your assistance in spreading the word about these offerings. The free book, Internet Resource Guide for Dementia Caregivers as well as Amazon links to the published paperbacks and eBooks are available through the website www.Caregiver10minuteguides.com.

And please contact me directly if I can assist further.

Sincerely,

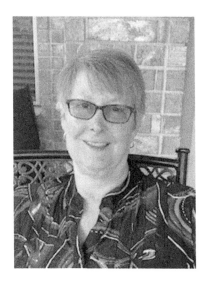

E. Jane Wyatt

M.A.; M.S.; Licensed Professional Counselor

CAREGIVER

Made in the USA
Las Vegas, NV
09 June 2023

73163106R00030